DON'T GIVE UP

A GUIDED JOURNAL FOR DEVELOPING AN ENTREPRENEURIAL MINDSET

RENA DAY

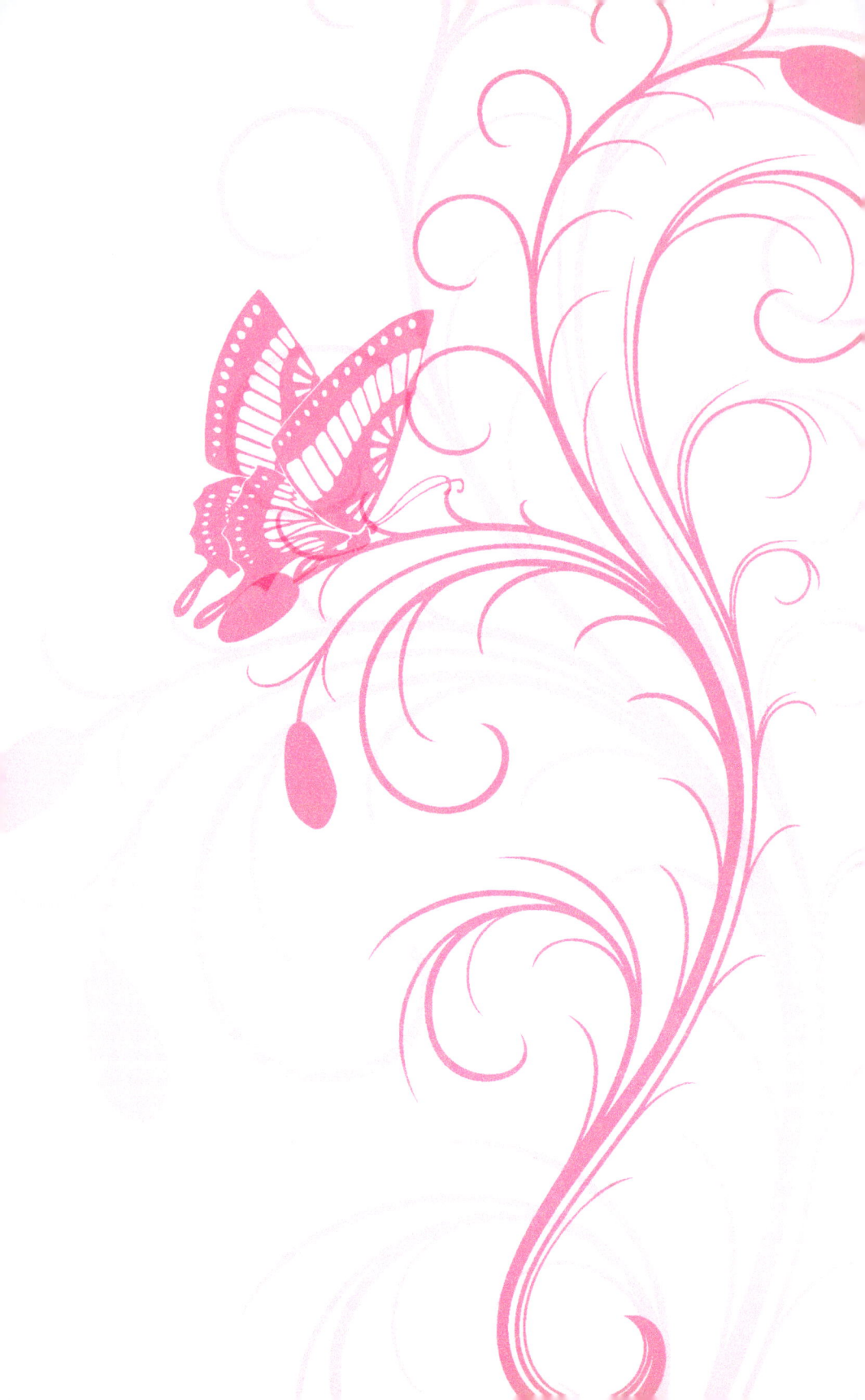

CONTENTS

INTRODUCTION 1

CHAPTER 1: DON'T GIVE UP 3

How To Overcome Obstacles 3

Don't Despise Your Humble Beginnings 5

Don't Lose Your Optimism 6

Let Expectations Be a Motivation But Don't Lose Sight of Reality. 8

You'll Never Know If You're Going The Right Way, So Just Keep Moving   9

CHAPTER 2: HOW TO KEEP GOING 11

Time Management 11

Delegate What You Can 13

Don't Overwork Yourself, But Work Hard 15

Fundraising/Investment Over Loans 17

CHAPTER 3: IT IS DARKEST BEFORE DAWN 21

Let Failure Be Your Stepping Stone 21

Rejection Is Good 22

Fear Is Your Enemy 23

Stress Is Crippling 25

Persist Through The Slump 25

CHAPTER 4: YOU CAN DO IT 27

Take Risks. 27

Work Harder Than Everyone Else 28

Build A Positive Reputation 30

Invest In Your Employees And Product 31

Celebrate Progress. 32

CHAPTER 5: THE MAKINGS OF SUCCESS 35

Be Bold And Decisive 35

Be A Master Of Improvisation. 36

Expose Yourself To New Opportunities. 37

Dream Big, Crazy, Scary dreams 38

CHAPTER 6: ENJOY THE JOURNEY 41

Have a Well Crafted Message 41

Enjoy Yourself 42

Don't Lose Your Identity 43

Be Authentic. 44

CONCLUSION 47

INTRODUCTION

Entrepreneurship is something so many people strive towards. Gone are the days when being an employee was the ultimate goal; more and more people are taking charge of their lives and diving into the deep waters of entrepreneurship with an exciting dream in their hearts that they are eager to share with the world, but then the harsh reality sets in and most of them shrink back into their shells and close themselves off for good.

You're probably reading this journal right now because you've lost hope and are ready to throw in the towel, or maybe you want to start but are too afraid to do so because you've heard a thousand horror stories about entrepreneurship. This journal will be the reason you don't give up.

There are so many reasons to give up but there are even more reasons to stick it out. Success won't come easy, and you will discover things along the way that might change the course of your business; the point is, don't give up. Keep your dream at the forefront at all times and you will always remember why you started when the urge to give up overwhelms you. The road to success is filled with great trials, but it is one that many have taken and arrived at the destination... And you can be one of those people too.

As you read this journal, I encourage you to take some time to seriously reflect on who you are, where you are and what you want to achieve. Self-awareness will not only make you successful but it will allow you to absorb the wisdom you will find in this journal and accurately translate it into your personal journey.

I wrote this journal because I know what failure is. I too have been there and felt a strong urge to give up and revert to my comfort zone where I was merely an employee working long hours for a monthly paycheck that would cover my bills. But when I remembered why I started, I was motivated to keep going.

Entrepreneurship can be a lonely journey, especially if you've been trying and failing. So, this journal is here to encourage and motivate you, as well as teach you what you need to know to turn your situation around. Most of the time we find that failure is the result of planting our seed in the wrong ground; the problem isn't with the seed itself.

This journal will teach you everything you need to know about entrepreneurship. It's highly possible that your past failures were a result of a lack of accurate information. Be open and honest with yourself while you read this and accept what you need to change. This may just be the journey that changes your life forever.

CHAPTER 1

DON'T GIVE UP

How To Overcome Obstacles

Obstacles are a part of life and will undoubtedly be part of your entrepreneurial journey. What will set you apart from those who have failed is how you handle these obstacles when you face them. Obstacles and entrepreneurship are synonymous with each other and you probably picked this journal up because you're faced with one.

To overcome your obstacles you need to be courageous, self-aware, determined, focused but most of all positive. What usually kills morale when one is faced with an obstacle is negativity. When you approach the situation from a negative perspective you are more likely to succumb to the pressure and give up. But when you look at the whole situation with a positive mindset, even if the situation itself isn't positive, you are more likely to find the solution.

Every entrepreneur needs courage in order to survive in this cutthroat arena. If you don't think you have the courage then you are wrong. The very fact that you chose to become an entrepreneur is proof that you are indeed courageous.

What you have to do is let go of your doubt and negative confession and you will find the inherent strength in yourself to keep fighting.

Secondly, you have to be self-aware. Successful people are usually the most self-aware because it takes a high level of consciousness of self to progress in life. You have to know your strengths and weaknesses otherwise you will never improve. Introspection should be a common task that you perform regularly to keep you grounded and focused. Being self-aware will help you accurately analyze your obstacles and allow you to determine the best course of action to overcome them based on your repertoire.

Thirdly, you have to be determined. Your situation won't change until you require it to change. Your determination will be the driving force behind your desire to overcome the obstacle you're facing and this is a result of your purpose. Don't forget why you started. Don't forget why you quit your job or invested your life's savings or sold your house; remember why you started. Remember everything that drove you away from being an employee to becoming an employer. When you keep the dream alive your determination and strong will remains strong.

And with determination comes focus. Focusing on what you want to achieve when you're faced with an obstacle is not easy. It is like being in the midst of a violent storm but visualizing on the destination instead of paying attention to the chaos around you. Having a solid focus will get you through a lot of things because it will force you to become creative. It will force you out of your comfort zone to find a solution because your mindset will be shifted away from your mapped out plan to alternative routes that will still get you to your destination.

Lastly, you need to maintain a positive mindset. This is obviously easier said than done, but fortunately, it is not impossible. Being positive is a conscious decision you have to make. It is something you have to work on and constantly be aware of. We often react to situations based on our subconscious, but when it comes to entrepreneurship you have to be mindful and alert whenever you're faced with an obstacle because you can unconsciously set a negative tone for your business, and no one is attracted to negativity so your business will not last under such conditions.

Don't Despise Your Humble Beginnings

It's easy to lose sight of your goal when you look at where you currently are and how little you have achieved. Discouragement creeps up on us so often because we have high expectations. It's normal and it's human.

Where you are right now in your journey is exactly where you need to be. This is just another step up the ladder to success. And while you are in that place your eyes should be peeled open for the lessons you need to learn, the skills you need to acquire and the improvements you can make.

Comparison will rob you of the joy of the experience but most importantly, it will rob you of your time. Judging your success by that of others is a sure way to fail. Think of your competitors as motivation and not as actual competition. By doing this you already eliminate the false narrative that you need to achieve what they have, to be considered as successful. The only way to determine true success is when you compare your current achievements to your dream.

Everyone has their own goals and dreams; therefore you cannot compare yourself to others. So don't look down on your current achievements because they pale in comparison to that of your competitors. You don't know what they had to go through to get to where they are therefore you cannot compare yourself to them.

Your main focus should always be yourself. Your business will thrive if you fix your eyes solely on it. In other words, all your attention and energy should be directed towards your business and away from what other entrepreneurs are doing or achieving. Yes, it is important to be aware of what others in the market are doing but don't compare yourself to them.

Where you are today is not where you will be in the next six months, but you have to acknowledge your position and work on improving it rather than sit in discouragement and stagnation.

Don't Lose Your Optimism

There will be times where you will feel like giving up; you will experience this more often than not, but this is when you need a visual reminder of the reason why you started.

Everyone knows who Bill Gates is and everyone wishes they were him or could at least achieve half of what he has, but no one talks about the struggles he went through to get to where he is today. In fact, most people only talk about his amazing achievements and yet Mr. Gates himself often reminds us that his journey was not easy. He often speaks about it because that is what made him one of the richest men in the world today.

Bill Gates is inspirational for his perseverance. No matter how many times he failed he remained optimistic that his Windows operating system would be operational and so he continued at it until he got a breakthrough.

What separates entrepreneurs like Bill Gates from the ones who fail is vision. When you have a vision and a conviction, that is all you will hold on to, and that is what fuels your optimism. Everyone who has ever invented anything will tell you that they tried and failed many times but they were optimistic because they had a vision.

Most businesses fail because the person with the vision lost sight of it or did not truly believe in it. In fact, numerous people start businesses with the hope of being successful but they don't really have a clear vision, but that's not you.

So the best thing to do for yourself is to write your vision and place it where you will see it at least once a day. Some people prefer to have a vision board instead which is even better because then you have a visual representation of what you see in your heart. By doing this you will constantly remind yourself of your end goal. When you feel like giving up you will have something to help you soldier on.

Failure is a part of life, but it is not meant to stop you, it is meant to teach and refine you. Besides, failure is relative. What may be considered a failure by the world can be considered a blessing to an individual. So, let failure just be another lesson to you.

There was a woman who quit her well-paying job to become an entrepreneur, and when asked what her expectation was of her business, her answer was, "I'm just trying something different and hoping it will work." Needless to say, her business failed and she went back to work a few months later. Why did this happen?

There are two sides to expectation; it's either you have a lot of it or you have none at all. In this woman's case, she had none. You cannot be an entrepreneur without expectation because this means you have no vision, and you cannot succeed without a sense of direction. The expectation is what motivates you to work towards your goals, so how then can you begin a business venture with no expectation at all?

Entrepreneurship isn't something you just have a go at; it is something that requires preparation, dedication, perseverance and hard work, therefore you cannot treat it like a game of chance where you just give it a try and hope you win. No! You have to actively pursue it with the belief that you will succeed no matter what.

On the other side of expectations are overly ambitious people. Some might say there's no such thing but there is. Some people would start a business today and expect to have massive returns within a month with no concrete plan on how they could possibly achieve that. Now, of course, this works for some people, but those are extremely rare and exceptional cases.

Yes, you have to be expectant; you have to expect success while you focus on reality. Dream big, but don't live in your dreams, instead work even harder to make your reality match your dreams because nothing will materialize if you don't put the work in. So don't get carried away by emotions and fantasies- and trust me you will experience this a lot- but live in reality because you might not be able to pick yourself up again if your expectation isn't met in the exact timeframe you desired.

So let expectation keep you up at night brainstorming new ideas, but don't let it overtake reality and destroy your dream.

You'll Never Know If You're Going The Right Way, So Just Keep Moving

There was a time before GPS' were introduced and one would have to use a map if you wanted to visit an unfamiliar area. You'd often get lost but still enjoy the journey because you discovered new places. That's what being an entrepreneur feels like.

When you are traveling on a road, you cannot see the entire length of the road but only the stretch that is within the confines of your vision, but you keep going because you believe you are headed in the right direction, and if an unexpected circumstance occurs along the way, you don't turn around and head back where you came from, instead you deal with the situation and carry on as best you can in those circumstances.

There's no way to accurately predict what lies ahead of you. You won't know what obstacles you will have to face, neither will you know the possible solutions you will have until you arrive at those obstacles. There is a high chance that you may have to take a different route than you originally intended but you just have to keep moving. The journey may differ but there will definitely be a destination, so don't lose sight of your goals just because things aren't going your way. Don't give up because you don't recognize your surroundings or your plan is rendered ineffective.

You will have doubts about whether or not you are headed in the right direction or doing the right thing, but the most important thing is that you keep going. Keep moving forward even if you aren't sure of your direction anymore because you will still arrive at a destination even if it isn't the one you originally intended.

We've all been taught in history that Christopher Columbus originally set out to find a direct route from Europe to Asia but instead stumbled upon the Americas. Even though he did not discover the Americas, he certainly became the bridge to the "New World". Unfortunately, he died with the impression that he had failed; completely ignorant of what he had indeed discovered.

You see, things will not always go your way and there will be times where you will have to alter your plans, or you may even make mistakes but all of this will lead you somewhere. It might be a happy accident and you arrive at your intended destination or it might be a completely different destination that holds greater returns, either way, you will always arrive at a destination.

CHAPTER 2

HOW TO KEEP GOING

Time Management

The initial stages of your business will be filled with a plethora of challenges to overcome and tasks to complete just to get the ball rolling and this can quickly become overwhelming if you don't manage your time correctly.

"Don't be fooled by the calendar. There are only as many days in the year as you make use of. One man gets only a week's value out of a year while another man gets a full year's value out of a week."
- Charles Richards

Time management is as important as planning and delegation. We all have 24 hours in a day; therefore we all have the same amount of time to achieve our goals. But what separates successful people from the unsuccessful ones is the ability to manage their time efficiently.

Good time management is about maximizing the time you have. This involves achieving as much as you possibly can within the same amount of time as everyone else. When you maximize your time you will achieve maximum results in return. In order to do this, you need to learn the principles of time management.

» **Have a concise plan** – Planning is good but strategic planning is even better. Plan exactly what you want to do, how you want to do it and the time you want to do it in.
» **Prioritize** – Work on tasks in order of importance.
» **Delegate** – Divide tasks amongst competent people who will get the job done within the desired time according to the given scope.
» **Be organized** – compartmentalize your tasks as much as you can because this will not only help in completing them but it will give you an accurate representation of your progress.
» **Be realistic** – Stick to what you know you can achieve before you strive for what you think you might. Ambition is good but over-ambition could cripple your business.

Time management is a vital skill that every entrepreneur needs to have in order to run a successful business. Life continues to move forward regardless of whether or not you move forward with it, so you have to make every minute as productive as possible.

Delegate What You Can

Most entrepreneurs fall into the trap of trying to do everything on their own. It is perfectly understandable because when you create something, you have a vision no one else will fully perceive so you try to do everything alone to get your desired outcome. Unfortunately, this may result in burnout, discouragement and maybe even physical illness.

The truth is that too many start-ups fail because the entrepreneur did not delegate. You cannot be everywhere at the same time and you cannot do everything by yourself either. It is impossible to build anything in isolation, so you have to ease off on the reigns a little and allow other people to help you; you have to trust other people and allow them to carry the burden with you.

You see, success is a result of a team effort. A team will always be more successful than an individual because a team comprises of a myriad of skills, talents, connections, etc. Whereas an individual can only produce what is in his or her own personal capacity.

Delegation is a difficult task, especially when you've tried and failed in the past or have been disappointed by people you trusted, but it is still something that must be done to build a strong, healthy business that will last. So you have to accept that delegation is one of the major factors that will guarantee longevity.

Bear in mind that delegation in itself is a skill. You have to have the wisdom to delegate correctly for you to obtain the maximum results. Intelligent delegation will make your business run like a well-oiled machine with all its parts functioning effectively thus producing the desired results.

So how do you delegate intelligently? There are certain traits and skills you should look for in your employees before assigning them to tasks and these are:

- » Work ethic
- » Skill level
- » Personality type
- » Leadership potential
- » Responsibility
- » Punctuality
- » Takes initiative
- » The ability to build a network
- » Strengths and weaknesses
- » Motive

The last point is especially important because anyone can be responsible, hardworking or any of the other traits listed but not everyone has the right motive. This is why it is vital that you truly understand your employees' characters before you entrust them with any form of leadership. The right people will be the ones who genuinely believe in your product or service and show commitment to wanting it to succeed. Such people can be identified by the way they represent your business in your absence. If a person truly believes in something, they represent it as if it is their own.

On the other hand, you will have employees who may have a bad attitude or are not committed to your company. Some might be jealous and not want you to succeed beyond a certain level while others may just have a bad attitude in general and not care about your business. Avoid giving such people power.

Anyone who is not as committed to growing the business as you are should not be a leader.

Another important thing to remember is to never promote people because of the length of time they've worked for you. Your business will not succeed on sentiment but hard work and dedication, so don't lead with emotion when it comes to delegation; think of who can get the job done most efficiently and effectively.

This doesn't always mean the most qualified person should be assigned the task; absolutely not. Most of the time, the people who know the most tend to deliver the least. This is because they are so pompous in their knowledge or credentials that they place more importance on themselves rather than the job at hand; so look for the person who is most committed to the business and allow room for them to learn and grow.

Delegating will be nerve-wracking until you build a solid trust, but it is necessary. You have to let go of fear, especially if you've experienced disappointment in the past, and trust yourself enough to make the right decisions on who to involve in your vision because the unfortunate truth is that you cannot do it alone.

Don't Overwork Yourself, But Work Hard

Being an entrepreneur requires a lot of time and hard work, and unfortunately this can land you in an endless cycle where you barely get any rest. We're living in a time where the importance of mental health has finally been recognized and acknowledged. It is indeed a large contributor to the success or failure of a lot of entrepreneurs.

Hard work surely pays, but you want to actually enjoy the fruit of your labor at the end of the day. You have to remember to do what is in the best interest of your health. This is also where delegation comes in. You can work hard but not be the only one working. Understand that hard work should aimed at a specific desired output; your job is to get the desired output not to look busy. It doesn't matter if two or ten people put in the work, what matters is that you get the output.

Therefore it is of utmost importance that your prioritize health. You can work hard but you have to set boundaries, not only for yourself but for your employees as well. So remember to delegate and manage your time well to create a positive work environment and allow you to lead a balanced life.

And don't be so hard on yourself if you don't get everything done according to your scope and time allocation. Instead, reassess your current operational plan to find where you can make changes that will benefit the business as well as its employees.

If you're just starting out and you happen to be the only "employee" you can still find alternative ways to get the job done efficiently that will allow you to rest. Don't be deceived into believing that working yourself to the bone is the only way to become successful. I'm sure you've heard many motivational talks in which the speaker tells you to work smart, well they're not wrong.

Fortunately, we live in a technological age; therefore there are a multitude of solutions that are available at our fingertips. Of course, this cannot completely substitute physical work but it can alleviate a lot of pressure and make everything easier and more efficient.

Fundraising/Investment Over Loans

The very first challenge most entrepreneurs face is funding. So many factors influence your ability to obtain funding especially from banks or lending institutions. If you've had a startup fail before you will understand how vital funding is but more importantly, how vital funding from the RIGHT source is. Yes, not all sources of funding are beneficial to your business. Now, this might sound strange to you but it is true.

There's a plethora of funding options out there, each with their unique terms and conditions. These terms and conditions have the ability to either build or break your business.

Now, you're probably wondering how funding can hurt your business, right? To determine this you have to know what sources of funding are available and what each one entails:

» **Yourself** – You should be the first person to invest in your business. This can be from savings or assets; even your time is a huge investment to your business. Investing in your business yourself gives you complete control over it, but unfortunately, failure means you lose everything you worked for.

» **Credit** – This includes loans from various institutions. The problem with credit is that you have to pay back the money with interest regardless of your business' success or failure. It also involves a qualifying criterion as well as a mountain of paperwork and you have to educate yourself in order to make an informed decision that will benefit your business.

» **Crowdfunding** – This is an umbrella term that includes other sources of funding such as family, friends, and donations, but the general idea remains the same. It is basically a group of people who give/donate money to your business. The investors usually don't require a return on investment which is good, but unfortunately, this will expose your ideas and plans to a large number of people which will make your business vulnerable to poachers (people who will steal your ideas and implement them while you amass funding).

» **Venture capital** – This type of funding comes from investors. It is great in terms of the exposure and credibility you immediately gain as well as the new networks and mentorship from the investors; however, you might lose a significant share of your business in equity to these investors as this is usually the only condition presented in exchange for capital.

» **Angels** – These kind of investors are very similar to venture capitalists in that they might require equity in exchange for capital, the only difference is that you may have to relinquish some control in some instances, but generally these are usually just wealthy people looking for something to invest in. You may be fortunate enough to find an investor who is knowledgeable in your field but you may also get the opposite. However, they usually provide more funding than venture capitalists which is a plus.

» **Government funding** – This is obviously funding obtained from the government. Unfortunately, there is usually a very strict qualifying criterion that you have to meet as well as adhere to certain terms and conditions. Bear in mind that government funding isn't available for every type of business so you will have to do adequate research to find out if there is funding available for your sector.

The best option when it comes to funding your business is yourself, and the best alternative is angel investors. But don't just find anyone with a ton of money at their disposal, you have to find someone who can truly understand the essence of your business and believe in it.

If you want to access funding that does not require a return on investment then you should go for crowdfunding options. Although this will require a lot of patience on your part because you might not arrive at the required amount in your expected timeframe. And remember to be cautious with this option because it involves convincing a large group of people to donate which means you might have to explain your business plan in detail.

Capital is always there, it just depends on where you look and what type of funding is best for you and your business. Just remember to be careful and not allow desperation to cloud your judgment because you might face terrible consequences down the road.

CHAPTER 3

IT IS DARKEST BEFORE DAWN

Let Failure Be Your Stepping Stone

I'm sure you know who genius inventor Thomas Edison is and are familiar with his story, particularly relating to the light bulb. While he was not the inventor of the light bulb, he invented the technology that made it commercial. The greatest part of this story isn't the invention, it's the 10,000 plus times he tried and failed. In fact, we cannot call them failures because Mr. Edison himself did not perceive them as such.

Now imagine all the people who probably ridiculed him or thought he'd never succeed with his invention; they had 10,000 reasons to believe it would fail, but Thomas Edison taught all of us a great lesson in that he didn't quit, he improvised. Each time his invention didn't work he changed something until it finally did.

Thomas Edison himself said, ***"I didn't fail 10,000 times. The light bulb was an invention with 10,000 steps."***

This is a very powerful statement. He let each "failure" be a stepping stone to his success. This is the same attitude that you need to have as an entrepreneur.

Your success is dependent on your inherent abilities. You might have to evolve with the times but don't allow change or the appearance of failure to distract you from your dreams. Choose to believe that failure is a lesson to be learned and not a destination to plant your roots.

Rejection Is Good

The business world is extremely competitive, therefore rejection is inevitable. In fact, rejection will be a very prominent aspect of your progress. This probably sounds crazy because no one would put rejection and success in the same boat, but it is a fact.

Every person who has ever achieved success has also experienced rejection at some point in their lives, but these people did not sit and soak in their rejection, instead they used that as motivation to push themselves harder than ever. As an entrepreneur, you must expect rejection because it will certainly come, but when it comes you have to be able to recognize the lessons and opportunities in it.

Rejection and failure are two of life's greatest teachers. Both of them possess the ability to refine you as well as your business. How shocked were you to find out that Steve Jobs, the genius founder of Apple was fired from his own company in 1985? You can imagine what he felt having been removed from something he birthed himself. But you see, no one can take your vision away from you, so don't pair rejection with failure because you carry the vision inside of you, so where you go it goes.

Use rejection as a time of reflection. Take the time to make the necessary changes to improve your product or service each time you hear a "no" until it is so good that it can no longer be denied. A lot of successful entrepreneurs will tell you that if they had never been rejected, they probably wouldn't have achieved their level of success.

Approval has a strange way of making us comfortable, whereas rejection forces us to improve. Every great leader, entrepreneur, politician, you name it, has a rejection story. This is because greatness is often birthed from rejection.

So when you are faced with rejection remember that it is good. Look for the lesson and/or opportunity presented in that "no" because your breakthrough might just be in it. Rejection may just be the right thing you need to push you out of your comfort zone and into greatness. So don't despise rejection, embrace it, learn from it and grow from it.

Fear Is Your Enemy

Fear is a part of life that no one can escape from. It is such a powerful force that will engulf you if you don't overcome it. The truth about fear is that it is a lie. It is merely a concept we construct in our minds due to unbelief in our own abilities.

The biggest fear many entrepreneurs have adopted is the fear of failure. When you think about it, they are actually afraid of something that hasn't happened yet, meaning they have visualized the possibilities and what they saw in their minds is what scares them, which isn't failure itself but the ridicule that comes from people.

Most of us are eager to try something over and over until we get it right, especially if it is something we enjoy, so how then can you be afraid of failing when you can get back up and try again? The problem is that fear has a way of magnifying everything, making it seem greater than it actually is.

My oldest sister taught me never to fear failure because I will fail at something eventually. So if I will inevitably fail at some point in life, why should I be afraid of failure? There is no human being who is perfect and capable of succeeding at everything they do, therefore you have to accept that you will fail, but that doesn't have to be your destination. (Remember failure is a lesson!)

Too many entrepreneurs give up halfway because of fear. In fact, some give up before they even begin because of fear.

"The graveyard is the richest place on earth because it is here that you will find all the hopes and dreams that were never fulfilled, the books that were never written, the songs that were never sung, the inventions that were never shared, the cures that were never discovered, all because someone was too afraid to take that first step, keep with the problem, or determined to carry out their dream."

- Les Brown

Fear will always be our greatest enemy because you can't win a battle if you've already defeated yourself in your mind. You need to make the conscious decision to fight against fear because you can conquer it. You can expose fear for the lie that it is and walk boldly towards your success.

Stress Is Crippling

Much like fear, stress has the ability to cripple us. Meaning it hinders us from making any real progress. But while fear is in the mind, stress affects the body. Physical illness makes us less productive in almost every area of life, and the unfortunate truth is that many life-threatening diseases are a result of stress. It hinders us from thinking rationally and performing to the best of our abilities; it alters our general behavior.

What you feel often bleeds into your business because it is an extension of you. If you are not feeling your best, the results will often appear in your business. Stress eats away at our lives and causes us to lose out on the enjoyment that comes from living. It also clouds your judgment and induces fear; so you are more likely to end up making rash decisions or ones based on emotion.

Some people believe that stress is the best motivator, but in actual fact, it is one of the quickest ways to kill your business. You won't always have it figured out, but adding stress to the mix is a sure way of inviting failure in. While it is possible to work under stressful conditions, it is not advisable to do so. It will kill your morale and create an unpleasant environment that won't produce the best results.

Persist Through The Slump

Like all good things, there comes a time where you will experience "the slump". You will feel hopeless, helpless, uninspired, discouraged and doubtful. It might even be made worse by stagnation in the business itself, which is usually when the urge to give up kicks in.

The slump is an unfortunate reality in everyone's life no matter what sector you fall under, but it's even worse as an entrepreneur. As an employee, all you have to worry about is getting yourself out of this dark place, but as a business owner everything rides on your shoulders, so you are responsible for your business' productivity, therefore you can't afford to be in a slump.

Here are a few things you can do to get yourself out of a slump:

» **Change your routine** – A slump is usually caused by routine. Once you are set in your ways there is usually a lack of motivation, therefore your mind and body begin to function on autopilot. So you need to shake things up a little.

» **Stimulate your mind** – This comes after changing your routine. Your mind needs to constantly be stimulated to be productive at a maximum level. To achieve this you need to find something creative and interesting to do.

» **Seek new ideas** – Sometimes all you need to get out of a slump is to do a little brainstorming. This, of course, should include other (trusted) people so that you can be refreshed by their unique perspective.

» **Take a break** – Every once in a while you need to rest. All you have to do is give your mind and body the time and space to reset and you will find yourself being refreshed and back to productivity in no time.

Don't beat yourself up when you experience a slump; instead, recognize that there is a change that needs to happen. Entrepreneurs are usually expected to function like robots and just keep working tirelessly, but you have to be kind to yourself as the leader, and your environment will respond in kind. It's okay to not always be at 100% but don't stay in your slump for too long otherwise you will fall into the trap of stagnation..

CHAPTER 4

YOU CAN DO IT

Take Risks

One of the greatest risk-takers who ever lived was Isaac Newton. He believed in his work so much that he was even willing to risk his life. Well, you don't have to be that dramatic, but you have to have that same passion.

Every innovator in history was a risk-taker. They went to lengths no one else would go despite being ridiculed and sometimes ostracized and plowed on with complete faith in their abilities and it paid off.

Every business owner has to take certain risks in order to grow. It may be scary and maybe even painful, but the risk is necessary for growth. Playing it safe might grant you success but it won't grant you longevity, and that's because the world around you is constantly changing as a result of someone else taking a risk. Just the fact that you took a risk to become an entrepreneur speaks volumes, but you have to continue on that trajectory.

You have to be cautious when it comes to taking risks. Yes, this sounds contradictory but you will soon realize that you cannot just take any risk; you have to take calculated risks. This means you have to approach the risk from various angles and try to determine the outcome from each, which would enable you to prepare a contingency plan in case of any unfavorable eventualities that may arise.

Therefore you should not just be a risk taker but a good risk-taker. You have to make informed, intelligent decisions to ensure that the risk you're taking produces favorable results. This means that you have to sharpen your critical thinking skills so you can accurately analyze the risk before you take it.

So don't be afraid of taking risks. If anything they should excite and motivate you because the presence of risk signals the presence of growth. Therefore the size of the risk will also determine the size of your growth.

Work Harder Than Everyone Else

This goes without saying; the hardest worker in your business should be yourself. Your vision, dream, and goals all began with you, therefore you have to be the one in the driver's seat steering your business in the right direction and controlling the speed.

Hard work is respected. Investors are more likely to invest in a business with a hardworking owner than one with a smart but lazy owner. That may not make sense but think of it this way, skills and intelligence can be acquired through learning, mentorship and life experience, but hard work is a choice. So what sets you apart from the next person is your work ethic.

People who work hard are the ones who get the job done. It's as simple as that. At the end of the day, investors, clients but most importantly yourself, want to see results. Of course, you have to exercise wisdom and intelligence but the most important thing is that you get the job done. Talking about what you can do or what you're going to do versus actually getting it done are very different things.

Startups have a fail rate of over 50% for many reasons- most of which you've read of in this journal. And you'll find that most of the ones who failed simply didn't work hard enough. Entrepreneurship is hard, so there is no room for laziness. You have to give it everything you've got if you're going to succeed. The level of hard work and dedication you put into your business will determine how others perceive it.

Remember, hard work isn't about how much physical effort you put into it, but it's about achieving maximum results in the allotted time. The best way to do this is to create systems that can operate independently while you work on what needs hands-on attention. These systems can include networks of delegated tasks or they can be technological, you can decide.

Your business will only grow as big as you allow it to. It is possible to stifle your growth due to laziness, so don't let yourself be the reason you fail. You have to find the courage and strength within you to push through the challenges and create something amazing.

Build A Positive Reputation

In the days of arranged marriages, families were very careful about their reputation. No one wanted to be associated with a family that had a bad reputation in the community. Therefore everyone was carefully intentional about the image they portrayed to the public.

Reputation is everything in the business world. Don't believe anyone who says things like, "All press is good press," because that is not true when it comes to business. I'm sure you know of at least one startup that failed due to bad publicity. People work very hard for their money and so they only want to spend it on what will be profitable to them.

Does it make sense to keep hiring a plumber who is terrible at his job? Absolutely not! The customer wants to get value for their money. Unfortunately, this one customer will also spread the word that plumbing company "ABC" provides terrible service, and thus no one will want to hire them.

Never underestimate the power of word of mouth. People tend to trust what they hear from someone with real-life experience of a particular product or service more than what is marketed to them in the media.

Because new businesses are popping up every day, you cannot afford to have a soiled reputation. You have to remain competitive in your niche by making sure you surpass the expectations of your clients. This means you have to be creative and innovative when it comes to your service offerings but most importantly, you have to provide value for money.

Always remember to respect your name; respect your business enough to want to keep it at a high standard. Also, respect your clients and their hard-earned money enough to meet their needs.

In your own experiences as a consumer of another business's products or services, you can agree that you won't settle for mediocrity, so you have to have the discipline and respect to uphold a certain standard as well.

Building a positive reputation will surely expand your clientele because everyone wants to be associated with excellence. Therefore always be intentional in every aspect of your business bearing in mind the consumer who is paramount to your success.

Invest In Your Employees And Product

Investment is vital for any business, but you have to realize that investment is not just a monetary injection into your business, it is also the skills and attributes you deposit into your employees as well as your business.

Employees are vital to every business. They are the driving force that propels the business forward. Therefore it is of utmost importance that you wisely invest in them. Your investment will not only be beneficial to their lives and wellbeing but it will be beneficial to your business especially.

Ways to invest in your employees:
- » Skills workshops
- » Teambuilding getaways
- » Better packages/ benefits
- » Flexible working hours
- » Good working conditions

For example, if your employees attend workshops regularly that expand their knowledge and skillset then you can add that to your business repertoire, therefore, expanding your clientele. So it's all about the bigger picture; what you put in is what you get out.

You also have to invest in your product or service. This means you have to refine what you offer. If it is a product, you have to make sure you source the best materials and labor which will enable you to produce an excellent product.

If you study marketing you will find that the most effective marketing tool is the product itself. What you produce will speak for itself, and your investment in it will determine whether it speaks positively or negatively. If you are providing a service, you have to invest in market research such as your competition and your target market, and use this information to refine your service to surpass your clients' expectations.

Celebrate Progress

Someone once told me a story of a businessman in Africa who died feeling disappointed because he did not achieve his lifelong dream of owning a shopping mall. He did, however, own a few stores in one of the major cities in his country, so he was by no means a poor man. The problem was that he was so focused on what he didn't achieve that he missed the joy in what he did. He never celebrated his achievements because they were not his original goal and died without truly grasping what he had actually achieved.

It is important that you celebrate every bit of progress along the way. It is better to take baby steps forward than to be stagnant. Not only does this boost your confidence but it is a constant reminder that you are headed in the right direction. The problem that many entrepreneurs have is that they don't celebrate their small victories. In fact, they don't even count these victories as progress because they seem insignificant. So many want that big break so badly that they miss the blessing that is in their small progressive steps.

It is better to have some progress than no progress. This may not be what you want to hear but it is the truth. Any type of progress is an indicator that you are doing something right, even if you don't realize it.

When you celebrate progress, you encourage yourself and the people who are working with you or the ones who have invested in you as well. This does not mean you should become complacent and lose your drive because you've made some progress, no, this should show you that you are capable of achieving your dreams even if it takes small steps instead of giant leaps.

When it is time for a baby to walk they start by crawling, then they learn how to balance on their feet, then they learn how to take a step or two, and finally, they can walk. Throughout this process, the parents celebrate every little progress the baby makes, and though the baby falls hundreds of times before they can actually walk, they get up and keep trying because someone is motivating them by cheering them on.

In your case as an entrepreneur, people might not celebrate your small steps of progress because it may seem insignificant to them, but you have to acknowledge what you have achieved and allow that to be yet another building block to your success.

When you learn to appreciate the little things you will have the confidence to aim for even greater things that will lead you to your end goal.

CHAPTER 5

THE MAKINGS OF SUCCESS

Be Bold And Decisive

We all have that one friend who can never make a decision when faced with options. These kinds of people can be frustrating and decelerating to progress. You cannot be one of these people. The success of your business relies on your ability to make bold decisions. Often times you might not have the luxury of time away to really assess the situation and plan before you decide and that is when you have to trust your gut and go for it.

Being bold means you should not leave any room for doubt; don't second guess yourself or try to imagine alternative possibilities, just make a choice and run with it. If you keep looking back, you might find yourself filled with the pain of regret of what could have been that it will cause you to live in the shadow of your past rather than the brightness of your future.

When you make those bold choices, resist the urge to revisit the past. Choose to keep looking forward without a glimpse of what could have been because the moment you look back you strip the choice you made of its boldness. Don't allow the "What if?" curiosity to rob you of the strides you've already made.

Cowardice and indecision will get you nowhere in life. You will find yourself running in circles thinking you are moving forward when the reality is you keep returning to your starting point over and over again. So you have to gain the courage to speak your mind and make your choices without fear and regret.

Be A Master Of Improvisation

Change is inevitable. This is one of the first lessons every entrepreneur needs to learn and accept because it will surely be required of you at some point. The harsh reality of life is that it is constantly changing and this change can either have a direct or indirect effect on you.

Sometimes you will face situations that are beyond your capacity; some might even leave you at a complete loss of what to do, where to go or who to ask. But instead of wallowing in negative feelings of failure, disappointment, and incapability, rather improvise. You have to have the ability to adapt to whatever situation you are faced with and that will require improvisation.

Take the Kangaroo rats for example. These are little creatures that have adapted to desert living by never drinking water and instead gaining the moisture they need from their food....

As an entrepreneur, you will face situations that will require you to adapt in order to succeed and this adaptation will require you to improvise with what you already have. Remember, don't change the essence of your business but you can tweak a few things that will enable you to move forward.

Adaptation does not mean changing the core of who you are as a person or the principals that your business is built on. It will never require you to lose your integrity. But you should welcome change and growth that will allow you to stay in your industry because change is often needed.

Expose Yourself To New Opportunities

Every entrepreneur has to have the ability to use their initiative. You have to constantly be on the hunt for new opportunities and insert yourself in spaces where these opportunities can find you.

I once asked a boutique owner if she had other stores around the city or even the country and her response baffled me. She said that expanding her business was not part of her plan; she was content with that one store because she didn't want the stress of owning multiple stores.

This is not the right mindset an entrepreneur should have. Growth and opportunity should always be something to strive for because if you don't grow you face the risk of being swallowed up by competitors. Looking around her boutique I found that there was nothing unique about her products so there was no reason to revisit her store when most of what she was selling was available at stores in closer proximity to my home, meaning she lost a client.

Don't be like this boutique owner! Don't limit yourself to your comfort zone because someone might even kick you out of it. There are probably thousands of other entrepreneurs trying to make it in the same market as you are, and let's be honest, all of you are in competition for the same clients.

This is why you have to be on the constant lookout for new opportunities and insert yourself in spaces that you normally wouldn't because you never know what you might find which could potentially alter the direction of your business and introduce you to new markets that you were unaware of.

To do this you have to keep your eyes and ears open at all times. Your opportunity may come from a client with unique needs to your product offering, or it could be an investor seeking to invest in a particular market field that you hadn't thought of but are capable of doing. Opportunities are literally everywhere just waiting for someone to notice and grab a hold of them.

Dream Big, Crazy, Scary dreams

It is time to stop playing it safe. There is so much that you achieve if you put fear aside, believe in yourself and just try. More often than not it is as simple as just giving it a try. Allow yourself to dream big; after all, you are the only one who can limit yourself.

Most entrepreneurs are comfortable but dissatisfied, and this is because they put limitations on what they could achieve and found no pleasure in it once they achieved their goals. There is no harm in having big dreams. The bigger, crazier and scarier they are the better. Having audacious dreams will keep you hungry and striving for more. You will never find yourself settling for a pit stop because you will always have the finish line in mind.

Don't let anyone dictate your life or how big your dreams should be. It is often the people without vision who have the most to say. You have to learn to drown out all the negative voices and focus on that dream that excites you and keeps you up at night. Don't be forced to live the life that everyone else is living because it is deemed to be more stable. Create your own path and go for what sets your bones on fire.

A dream is not meant to reflect reality anyway, so don't hold back because others cannot see what you see. It will sound crazy to a lot of people but just take comfort in the knowledge that it wasn't meant for them in the first place therefore their opinions cannot define your dreams.

CHAPTER 6

ENJOY THE JOURNEY

Have a Well Crafted Message

A lot of your initial struggles can be sorted by having a well-crafted message. What is it that you're trying to communicate to the consumer and how effective is it?

A well-crafted message should be simple, alluring and honest but most of all it should have direction. This means it should have a clear target market. Hundreds of businesses fail because they don't have a clear vision, target market, and message, therefore they cannot communicate effectively to meet the consumer's needs.

This is one of the most important things you have to think about when drawing up your business plan. A successful entrepreneur is one who meets a specific need, so your message has to reflect your desire and ability to meet that need.

So don't give up if you're not getting enough clients, instead reevaluate your message; reevaluate what you have to offer and if the message you are communicating accurately describes the service you're offering and how that message is perceived by consumers.

There have been a number of products that have been discontinued over time, not because they were ineffective but because they were not clearly communicated to the consumer, neither were they directed at the right target market. When you know and understand your message, you will understand exactly who needs to hear it, thus ensuring success.

For example, musical artists often begin their careers with a very specific audience in mind and they tailor their performances to meet the expectations of their audience. As their audience increases, they gain more and more room to switch things up and branch out into other genres.

That is how you should approach business as well. Have your niche and stick to it until you have solidified your place in the market and can afford to try new things.

Enjoy Yourself

Entrepreneurship will require a lot from you and unfortunately, you cannot escape challenges. But in the middle of it all, will be the most amazing experience of your life and someday you will look back on it all and marvel at the journey more than the destination.

Work harder than you ever have in your life but don't forget to enjoy yourself. Yes, it will be difficult and you will have to endure many things in order to succeed but you will find it enjoyable and fulfilling because you would have done what many have failed to do and gone where many have failed to go. You will look back at every obstacle you had to overcome and the fears you had to defeat to achieve your dreams and it will all be worth it.

And even though the journey is filled with ups and downs, it is also filled with precious memories that you will be the making of the legacy you leave for future generations. Someday you will look back and remember where you began with every rejection, failure, obstacle, fear, expectation, hard work, risk, investment, and decision and you will probably wish you had started sooner so you could enjoy it longer.

So don't be so focused on the destination that you miss the beauty that is in the journey. Some day you could be the multimillionaire that everyone invites to speak. You have the potential to be the next world changer, so live in the present as much as you imagine your future and revel in the experience.

Don't Lose Your Identity

Who am I?

This is a question every person needs to ask themselves.

Identity is a big struggle for so many people and rightly so. Your identity is the core of who you are as a person and everything you do flows from that. It is even more important to know and understand your identity as an entrepreneur as well as the identity of your business because that is how you will identify your market.

It is important to not only know who you are but to stay true to who you are. There will be instances where you will be tested and your identity will be threatened, but when you understand who you are, you will not be shaken.

Many startups have quickly been bought out by big investors or corporations and turned into huge successes because these investors understood the identity of the business and/or product and therefore saw its true potential. Of course, it may be beneficial to sell when the offer arises but before you make such a decision you need to understand the true identity of your business.

Sometimes we get so caught up in all the ruckus that we lose sight of what it is that makes our business special, therefore undervaluing it. When you lose your identity, you lose your authenticity and merely become a shadow of your former glory. So don't ever take anything for granted no matter how successful you become. Don't ever lose the essence of your business. Don't ever lose yourself.

Be Authentic

Be true to yourself. You may receive criticism and rejection, but remain true to yourself and your business/product. No one can believe in your business more than you can, and no one can understand your vision better than you can.

Think of counterfeit goods. They may look like the original but they don't possess the same quality, therefore, they don't last as long as the original product and in the end, people would rather spend more on the original and receive better quality and functionality than spend less on a counterfeit that won't last.

Despite what people say, your product or service is valid and those who don't understand it are simply not your target market. It's easier to focus on the naysayers because their voices are usually the loudest but don't let them deter you from your mission.

Those who cannot see your vision will be the most opinionated but you have a choice on what to believe and what to accept. If you feed on that negativity it will yield negative results, but if you focus on your dream and stay on track you will surely prove them wrong.

Improve your business but don't alter the vision. The process may change along the way because life is full of unexpected occurrences that require you prove your flexibility and readiness for change.

At the end of the day, people are drawn to authenticity. Consumers will trust, respect and recommend what they trust and believe in. Authenticity will guarantee longevity.

CONCLUSION

I hope this journal shifted something within you and ignited a new fire to aggressively go after your dreams. I hope you were encouraged, but most importantly I hope you learned new lessons that will be beneficial to you for years to come.

Russell Conwell delivered a speech entitled "Acres of Diamonds" in which a man named Ali Hafed sold his farm and went in search of diamonds. He traveled far and wide until he lost all he had and committed suicide because of the shame of returning home empty-handed. The sad part of this story was that the new farm owner discovered the diamonds on the very farm Ali had sold to him and it so happened to be what we know as the diamond mine of Golconda. I recommend you read or listen to the full speech so you can grasp the weight of this story.

All this is to say that you should not be hasty to chase after the success that you've only heard stories about. Focus on your own journey and your own dreams and ignore what everyone else is doing or saying because more often than not our breakthrough is much closer than we think, but we miss it because we are so focused on what we cannot see.

You may have an idea that you don't think is good enough so you focus on finding what you think will appeal to the masses instead of being bold, taking a risk and refining your idea to appeal to the masses. There is only so much that you can do in a lifetime, so focus on what you have the vision and ability to do and there you will find your success.

THIS JOURNAL BELONGS TO

MY DECLARATION

This Year, I Am Going To:

I Will Achieve This By:

I Might Need Help With:

I Know I Can Complete This By:

MONTH
1

YOU'LL NEVER KNOW IF YOU'RE GOING THE RIGHT WAY, SO JUST KEEP MOVING.

NOTES

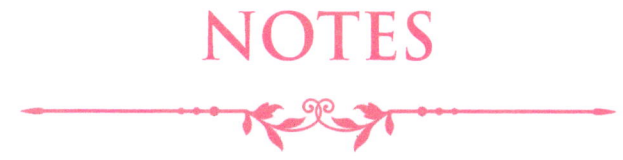

How was your month? What did you achieve?

What can you improve? How do you feel?

MONTH
2

DON'T OVERWORK YOURSELF, BUT WORK HARD!

NOTES

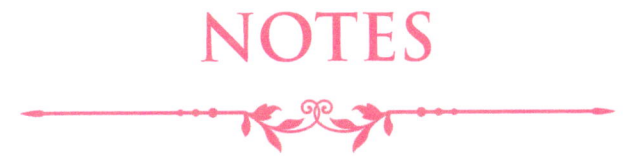

How was your month? What did you achieve?

What can you improve? How do you feel?

_____

_____

_____

_____

_____

_____

MONTH

3

LET FAILURE BE YOUR STEPPING STONE

NOTES

How was your month? What did you achieve?

What can you improve? How do you feel?

MONTH

4

JUDGING YOUR SUCCESS BY THAT OF OTHERS IS A SURE WAY TO FAIL!

NOTES

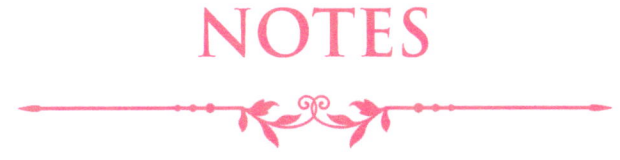

How was your month? What did you achieve?

What can you improve? How do you feel?

_____

_____

_____

_____

_____

_____

MONTH

5

WE ALL HAVE 24 HOURS IN A DAY TO ACHIEVE OUR GOALS... USE YOURS WISELY!

NOTES

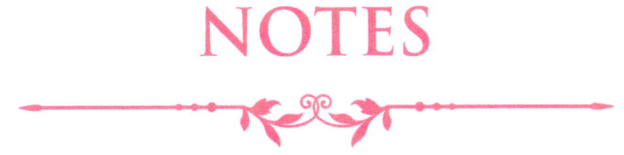

DATE :

How was your month? What did you achieve?

What can you improve? How do you feel?

MONTH
6

PRIORITIZE YOUR MENTAL, PHYSICAL AND SPIRITUAL WELL-BEING!

NOTES

How was your month? What did you achieve?

What can you improve? How do you feel?

MONTH
7

FAILURE IS A LESSON TO BE LEARNED, NOT A DESTINATION TO PLANT YOUR ROOTS!

NOTES

How was your month? What did you achieve?

What can you improve? How do you feel?

MONTH
8

REJECTION AND FAILURE ARE TWO OF LIFE'S GREATEST TEACHERS!

NOTES

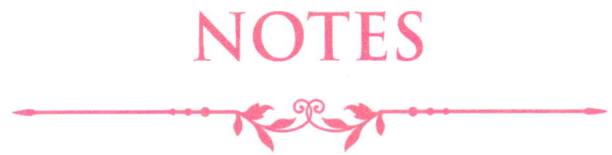

How was your month? What did you achieve?

What can you improve? How do you feel?

_____

_____

_____

_____

_____

_____

MONTH
9

PROGRESS IS PROGRESS NO MATTER HOW SMALL!

NOTES

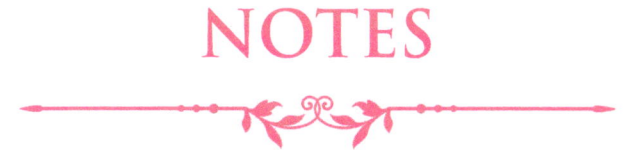

How was your month? What did you achieve?

What can you improve? How do you feel?

_____

_____

_____

_____

_____

_____

_____

MONTH
10

THE SUCCESS OF YOUR BUSINESS RELIES ON YOUR ABILITY TO MAKE BOLD DECISIONS!

NOTES

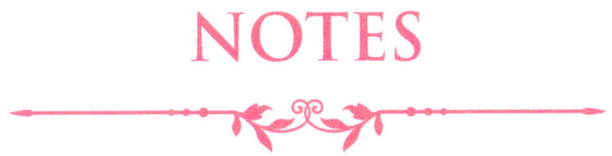

How was your month? What did you achieve?

What can you improve? How do you feel?

_____

_____

_____

_____

_____

_____

MONTH
11

DON'T LIMIT YOURSELF TO YOUR COMFORT ZONE BECAUSE SOMEONE MIGHT KICK YOU RIGHT OUT OF IT!

NOTES

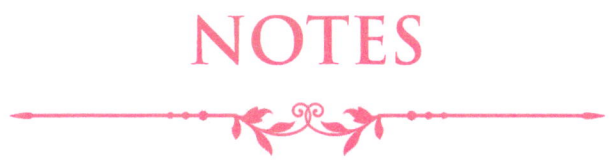

How was your month? What did you achieve?

What can you improve? How do you feel?

MONTH
12

DON'T BE SO FOCUSED ON THE DESTINATION THAT YOU MISS THE BEAUTY OF THE JOURNEY!

NOTES

How was your month? What did you achieve?

What can you improve? How do you feel?

CPSIA information can be obtained
at www.ICGtesting.com
Printed in the USA
BVHW021039220520
580137BV00013B/135

9 780578 679501